Closed For Now

A Pandemic Experience

Frank Prem

Wild Arancini Press
2026

Publication Details

Title: Closed For Now: A Pandemic Experience
ISBN: 978–1–925963–13–7 (p–bk)
ISBN: 978–1–923166–35–6 (e–bk)

Published by Wild Arancini Press

A catalogue record for this book is available from the National Library of Australia.

Disclaimer: This is a work of creative non-fiction, based on real events as encountered by the author through direct experience, observation, or in response to media reportage. Some names, places, and identifying details have been changed to protect privacy and maintain anonymity. Certain characteristics such as occupations, physical descriptions, and places of residence may also have been altered.

Please note: this poetry collection may contain occasional coarse language.

"Unknowing (the City)" was first published in This Is Lockdown: COVID19 Diaries Flash Fiction Poetry, edited by M.J. Mallon – Kyrosmagica Publishing (2020).

Images used in this book are photographs of shop signs displayed in Beechworth, Victoria during the Covid lockdowns of 2020–21, taken by the author using a phone camera.

Cover concept: Wild Arancini Press
Cover image AI assistant: Adobe Firefly

Which of us knew, back then, that this was war?

CONTENTS

Closed For Now

After Words

Closed For Now

Introduction

The year 2020 seemed to mark a nightmare awakening in a shockingly brutal reminder of the consequences of humanity's presence on the Earth.

In Australia it began with vast tracts of land burning at the uncontrollable whim of wildfire. The scale of destruction, the loss of wildlife and habitat, and the human cost were catastrophic beyond description. It is a deep sadness to recognise that many other parts of the world have since burned just as fiercely, each in their turn.

By February of that year, another scourge was spreading across the globe. Coronavirus (COVID-19) swept through communities like a tidal wave, its deadly potential revealed everywhere.

It was during that first wave of Covid here in Victoria, Australia, that the poetry in these pages was written.

Closed for Now is a poetry collection in two parts.

The first section captures the early experience of the pandemic – as it was lived, reported, and witnessed. It speaks of people thrown out of work, paralysed by sudden fear, and of others lashing out in anger or confusion, using accusation and assault as a way of coping with the unknown for which none of us were prepared.

The second section of the book, titled *The Facility*, tells the story of an elderly person passing away in residential care – a nursing home – during those uncertain first months.

This is poetry of experience: bitter, raw, and immediate. A reflection of the strange new reality of our times – the lived pandemic.

Part I: Closed For Now

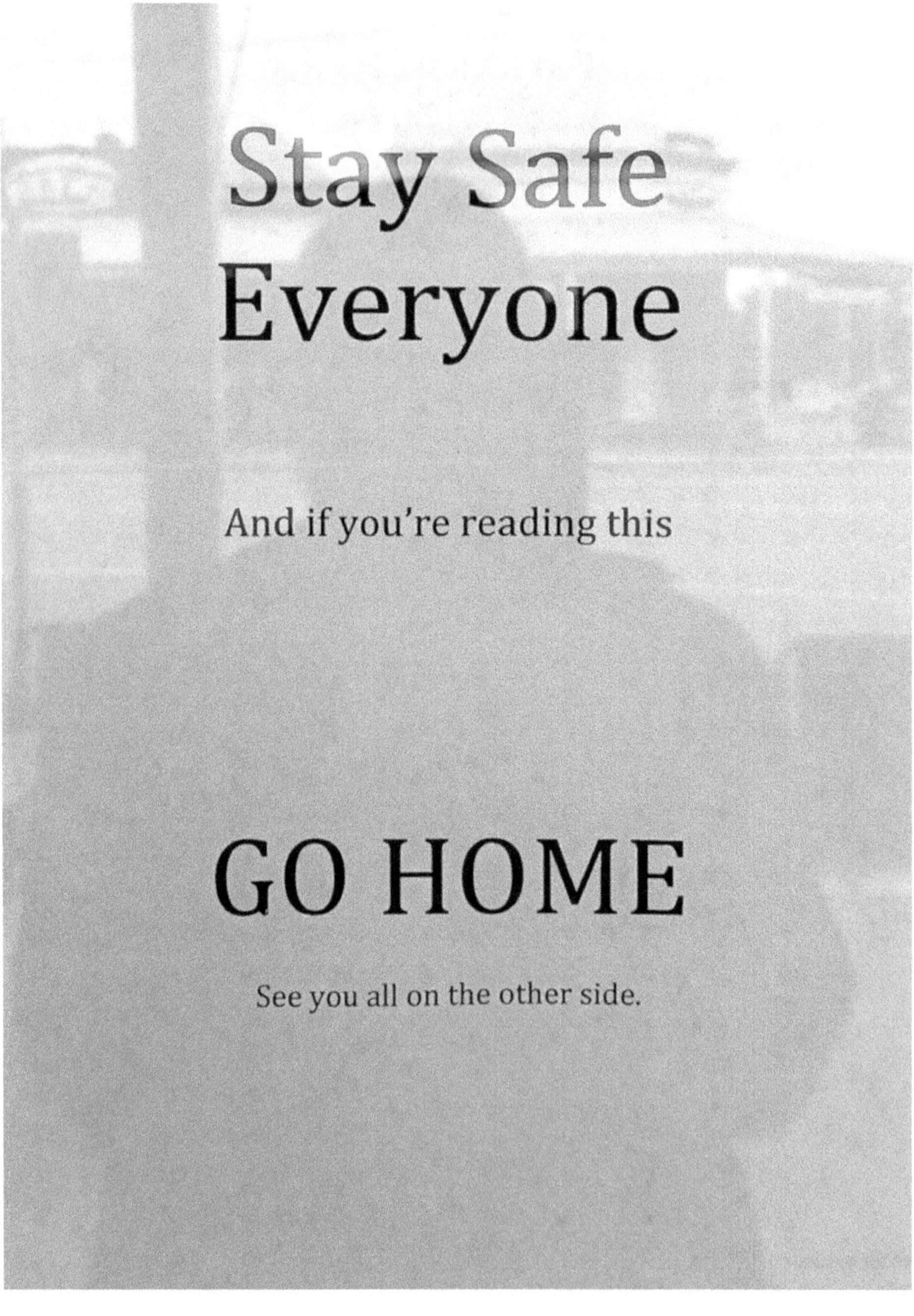
Stay Safe
Everyone
And if you're reading this
GO HOME
See you all on the other side.

covid (I don't think so)

did you hear . . .

can you
believe it . . .

surely
it can't
be true

they're closing
all the libraries

shutting down
the schools

trying
to cordon off
the airports

to make sure no virus
can walk through

a new section
of the newspaper
is titled *corona*

covid
number nineteen

and already
I think I hate it

I think it
a loathsome thing

did we not have
enough
to get through
without this panic
of the plague

and I wish . . .

you *know*
I wish . . .

. . . wish I could believe
there is anyone
that knows
what the hell to do

but
somehow

I don't think so

a fingertip away (from switzerland)

I took a moment
to google
this

the earth

I started out
somewhere
above switzerland

then africa

found antarctica
before I got to australia

tasmania

and the blue
of the oceans deep
was a meditation
passing

the green
of the forests
was a cry
that I felt as though
the beating
of my own heart

and I wondered
if they have
the colour
wrong

if maybe
a new photo
would show
black
after the fires

it's a small world
when you can push it
around
using just the tip
of a single finger

I use a flat screen
for my trans-global
navigations
but
I can imagine it
as a globe

spinning

as I
am spinning

from the *lockdown*
of a little room
with everything else
out there

away
out there
while the world
is contained
within a solitary mobile phone

and I think
I should turn it off
right now

there is a virus
running wild

and the distance
(as I know now)
between switzerland

and the antarctic

and tasmania

and me
is very small

is just
one tiny touch
of a fingertip
away

from quarantine room three (I call home)

will we have
love

here
in room three

I think I saw *you*
entering
room four

but
the door is closed

the way
is shut

I can only wonder
my thoughts of you
by myself

we could not
be
together

it was said
that we
had to bear this load
alone

and *that*
it seems
makes the weight
much heavier

there is no one
to keep me
from thinking

(from feeling)

of the small harms
perhaps
about to befall me

are they falling
on you

knock knock

tap

rap
tap tap

knock knock

are you at home

like
I am
in this *room three*
that I
call my own

I'll see you
in a fortnight

I'll see you
in a dream

I'll see you in my mind
each time
I lean my body
against the wall
that runs between us

catch me
in your thoughts

in *room four*

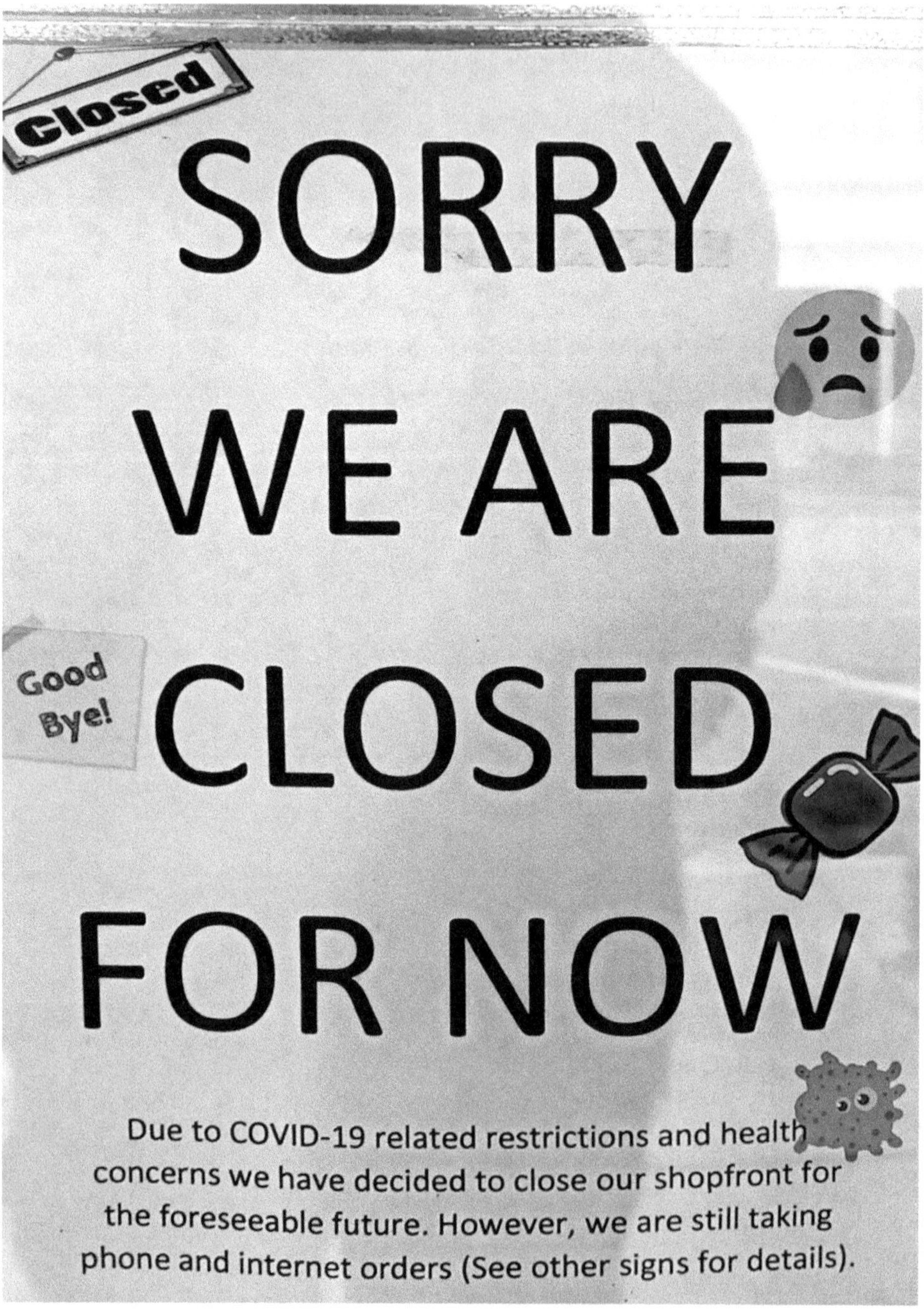
Closed
SORRY
WE ARE
Good Bye!
CLOSED
FOR NOW
Due to COVID-19 related restrictions and health concerns we have decided to close our shopfront for the foreseeable future. However, we are still taking phone and internet orders (See other signs for details).

better off (don't touch me)

and every day
I wake
and wonder

have I
caught
a cold

my throat
feels tight
the back of my head
seems nasal

cough

I splutter
a little . . .

sort of
experimentally

I want to get a sense
of whether I *rasp*
or
if I sound
ok

and I place my hand –
the back
of my hand –
against
my forehead

I'm not supposed
to touch myself
but the back of a hand
seems acceptable

and I badly want
to be reassured
that I don't have
a fever

I guess
I'll wash my hands
again
when I get up
out of bed

there's no hope
for me to stay
clean
the way they want me to
and
I know it

the habits
of a lifetime
will likely kill me
if I go outside

or at least . . .

at least
they'll get me quarantined

so
a fist bump (*no*)
maybe

an elbow (*yes that's better*)

or
I could crash into you
with a *hip-and-shoulder* charge
just to say

hi

hello

but more likely
I'm going
to touch you

I won't mean to
of course
but we both know
that's just the way
that I am

we will be better off
it seems
if I stay
isolated

better off
and maybe . . .

just *maybe*

unharmed

popcorn endings (alright?)

do you remember
the days
we used to make
popcorn

add a bit of butter
to the pan

heat it up

throw in the kernels

put the lid on

not many seconds gone
and they'd start
banging away

then
we would watch
a movie
on tv
in the quiet

we had a dog then

she had a nose
for popcorn
and other treats

one for you
one for me
one
for the dog
that made us *three*

everything is different
now
and I'm stuck
at home

the tv is running
on the news
twenty hours
in the day

I've got cans
of food

and toilet paper

pasta
at the ready
should I feel the need

but
what I really miss

the thing I want
is popcorn
in a big bowl
while I watch
the world unformed
like
in a movie

a great big
disaster movie

I could pretend
to myself that
maybe
by the time I reach
the bottom of the bowl
it will end alright

I wish
that I knew
it would end
alright

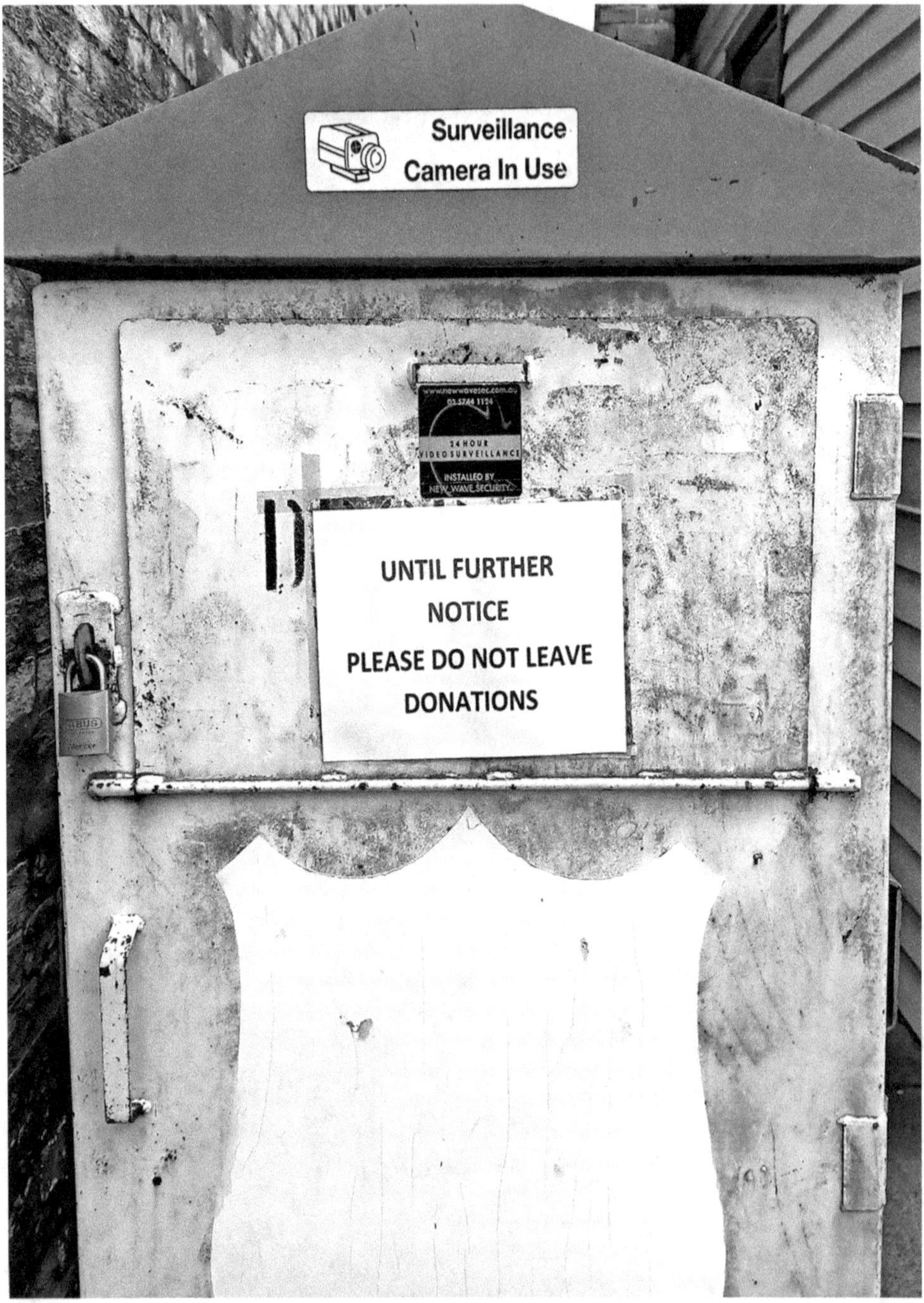
Surveillance
Camera In Use
24 HOUR
VIDEO SURVEILLANCE
INSTALLED BY
NEW WAVE SECURITY
UNTIL FURTHER
NOTICE
PLEASE DO NOT LEAVE
DONATIONS

trying to find it (only in the quiet)

I've looked hard
all around me
to try to spot
the change

but
I get nothing
until I see the newspaper
lying open

there it is
in big bold print

and
there it is
written up
as fact

when I look up
again
it hovers
in the air
before fading

and I blink
like a man
who has been
sleeping

everything around me
seems right
but
a touch surreal

so
I look again

see nothing
this time

I search
into every corner

but it is only
when I *see* the tv set
that it starts
blaring

and I feel myself
filling up
with *corona*

I feel myself
leaking it
from every pore

thank god
for the press
thank god
for the anchor-folk
on the all-day news broadcasts
for not stopping

not even long enough
to breathe the air
of *covid*

covid-19

maybe
to inhale –
just once –
might herald
the end
a little prematurely

because
there is so much to say
so much
analysing
to do

let them
hold their breaths
while they talk
and talk
forever

there is something new
each moment
to be concocted

or fantasised

but I think
just now
I'm going to burn
the newspaper

turn the tv off
and see
how I feel
when it is
quiet

I thank god
for quiet

early opening (and much better off)

she said

they opened
the grocery shop
an hour early

so people like me –

the old and frail
and
the disabled –

could get our things
before the panic buyers
descended

that
was nice
of them

very *nice*
of them

there were empty
shelves
in the toilet paper
aisle

just one stray box left
of oversized
and overpriced
tissues

I couldn't get
a thing
that I
really needed

she said

it was very lovely
of them

to open up
for me
but . . .

what was the point

I'm wondering
if there was
any point at all

I would have been
better
to stay at home

maybe
it would be
better
if I die

if people
like me
just die

there is nothing
in the grocery shop
for me

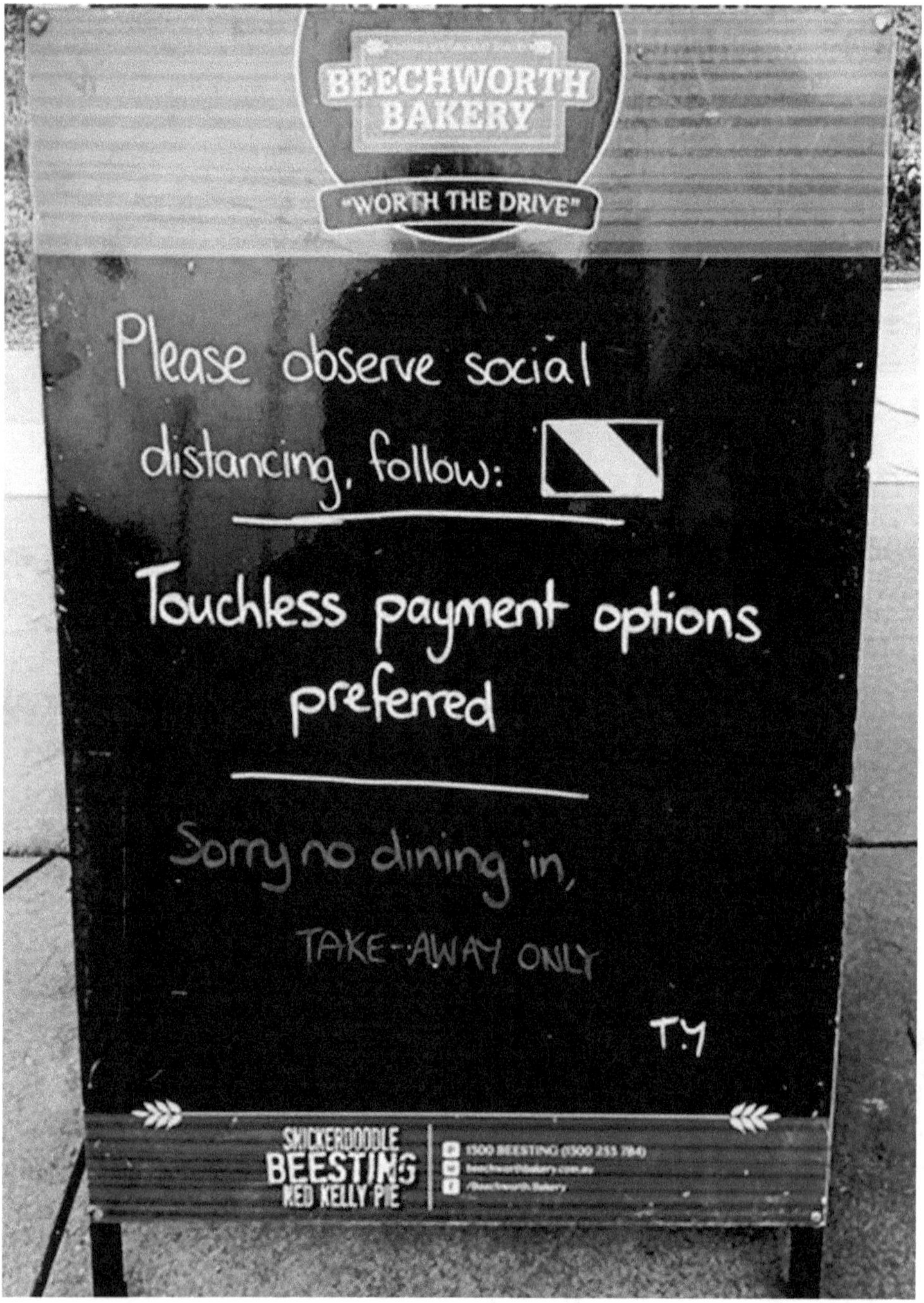
BEECHWORTH
BAKERY
"WORTH THE DRIVE"
Please observe social
distancing, follow:
Touchless payment options
preferred
Sorry no dining in,
TAKE-AWAY ONLY
T.Y
SNICKERDOODLE
BEESTING
RED KELLY PIE

a pity (in a drowning)

the stock market died
a little bit more
today

I think it died
from an even bigger fall
yesterday

I used to think –
once
upon a time –
that you work through your life
and then retire

little by little
that truth
has gone
like the breath
of a politician's promise

the pension
was supposed to be there
for older folk
at the end
of their toiling life

a little payback
for being
a good citizen

but then
they brought in
superannuation
to keep us
better
in our old age

and little by little
the pension
has become
a small way further off . . .

into the future

reserved now
for the
really old

they say
that someone like *me*
is supposed to be ok
with just
their superannuation

you know
all those *superior* earnings
from sound investment
in stocks and bonds

all made by smarter men
and women
than *I* am

than I
will *ever* be . . .

but the market died
for the fourth time
in a week

it's started
to resemble
an ashpit
of dreams that burned

of hopes
that couldn't outlast
the fire

just bad luck –
I guess –
on top of bad luck

Closed For Now

I’m not sure
what I’ll do now
to make ends meet
if this virus
ever slows down

if no fires
ever start up again

and if the gods
don’t take
a little cruel pity
and just let us
drown

stella's song: getting by (on plastic)

I live
on the welfare line

get my money
through a plastic card

no gambling
and no
alcohol allowed

but if my shop
happens to sell
beer
or those scratch-ie lottery cards
then my welfare plastic
is no good there

I live
in a little town

not much choice
about
where I can go

now
they're going to put me
into quarantine

some kind of self-isolation

and they'll pay me
a little bonus
(or
at least
they'll pay it
to my plastic)
to see me through
this hardship time

Closed For Now

that's nice of them

this government
is kind

but
the only shop in town
(that sells
no alcohol
and
no lottery cards)
has run out
of groceries

and I can't use the bonus
to wipe
my sorry arse

or eat
a can of
governmental
good intentions

I've got
a couple of packets
of potato chips

some doughy bread

runny butter

and chicken nuggets
in the back
of the freezer

I live
very small

and I guess
that I'll survive it

happy birthday (twice) to me and you

I am singing
happy birthday
to me

I am singing it
again
from start
to end

singing a little song
like *happy birthday*
can make me safe
if I use the soap
and rub my hands
scrub myself
clean
while I sing it

it isn't *really*
my birthday . . .

I suppose you already knew

this is just a way
to learn

they tell me
if I sing
the
happy birthday song
nice and slow
while I wash my hands
I might live
to see another birthday
down the road

so sing with me

happy birthday
to you

and sing

happy birthday
to you

(that's twice)

I'll see you
in a while
when your . . .

when *my*
birthday comes around

and I'll sing
happy birthday twice
(again)
with you

a hen (or four)

it's hard to say
for sure
but
we may get
a hen
(or four)

to run
with our new
garden beds . . .

our vegetables
and the fruit

we've often
wondered
about getting chooks
but

> *will we be here*
> *to look after them*

always
that has been
the question

right *now*
we're being
here
quite a lot

so
maybe
a hen would be ok
(or four)

perhaps
this
is the time

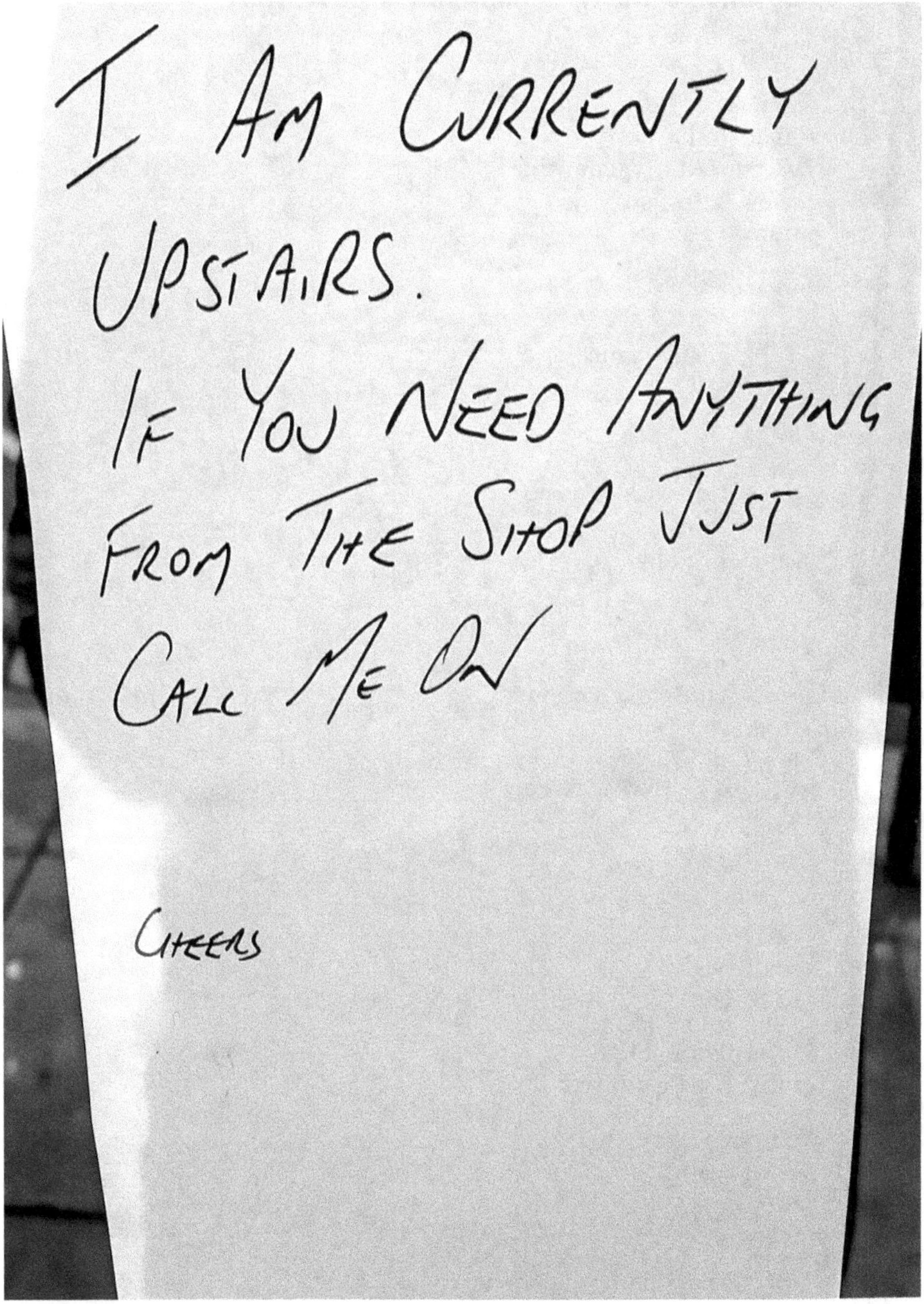
I AM CURRENTLY
UPSTAIRS.
IF YOU NEED ANYTHING
FROM THE SHOP JUST
CALL ME ON
CHEERS

no-one to watch it happen (in australia)

well
in australia
we started to quarantine
a few years ago
now

we called it

border control

and

turn back the boats

said things like

we control
who
gets into this country

it was almost
a novelty
back then

~

no one
is allowed
to fly away

international lines
must not be crossed

every country
is an island
now

but I can still wave
to you
across an ocean

shore to shore

until they stop us

~

there are dolphins –
or
so I've heard –
swimming in the canals
in venice

probably just a story
but they say
that there is so little
humanity
moving around over there
that the water
has become clear

clean again

sometimes
the image
of a city street
is just a picture
of the people on it

a sea of heads bobbing
as a kind of strata
of shifting bodies

but now the picture
everywhere
is visible architecture

empty roadways
like a post-apocalyptic
abandonment

I hear my own feet
as they scuffle
along empty roadways
and pavements

~

tonight
I watched
a football game
on the tv

it was strange

players on the field
umpires
to do the refereeing
and

no-one else

except
security guards
to keep the people out
who would *otherwise*
have come in

no fans at all
today

their noise
audibly replaced
by every call
and every curse . . .

every spit
onto the ground . . .

by
all the umpire's
explanations . . .

I missed the *roar*

that great upwelling
of sound
when a goal
was scored

the commentary team
spoke in turns
exercising
a professional
social distancing

about
a metre and a half
is what it sounded like

and they called the game
as if
it was football
but . . .

it didn't really
feel
and it didn't
really *look*

didn't really *sound*
like anything more
than desperation
and
denial

my team lost

and I think
my team
always will

in lonely defeats
by an implacable
foe

and nobody
will be allowed
to catch an aeroplane

or to land
ever again
in australia
to watch it happen

mask (and demise)

driving through
a little town
today

I saw someone –
a student
from a local school –
walking on the small
main street

wearing a face mask

imagine . . .

masks
worn casually on the street
in the daytime

it's still
an unusual sight
where I live

they catch
the attention

~

an article
on the newsfeed
today
described an assault

down south of here
in tasmania

a man
of asian appearance
and
wearing a mask
was punched

a blow to the head

accused –
in an abusive tirade –
of *conspiracy*

of deliberately bringing
the virus plague
to our shores

it was
stupid

and
it was personal

~

who are
the australian people

I mean
who are we
on the inside of ourselves
when the chips
are down

paranoid denialists

xenophobic
finger pointers

self-serving
hoarders
of toilet tissue
and daily detritus

helpless
in the face
of challenge

brittle and shallow
naïve
and foolish

and open

so
wide
open

to our own
demise

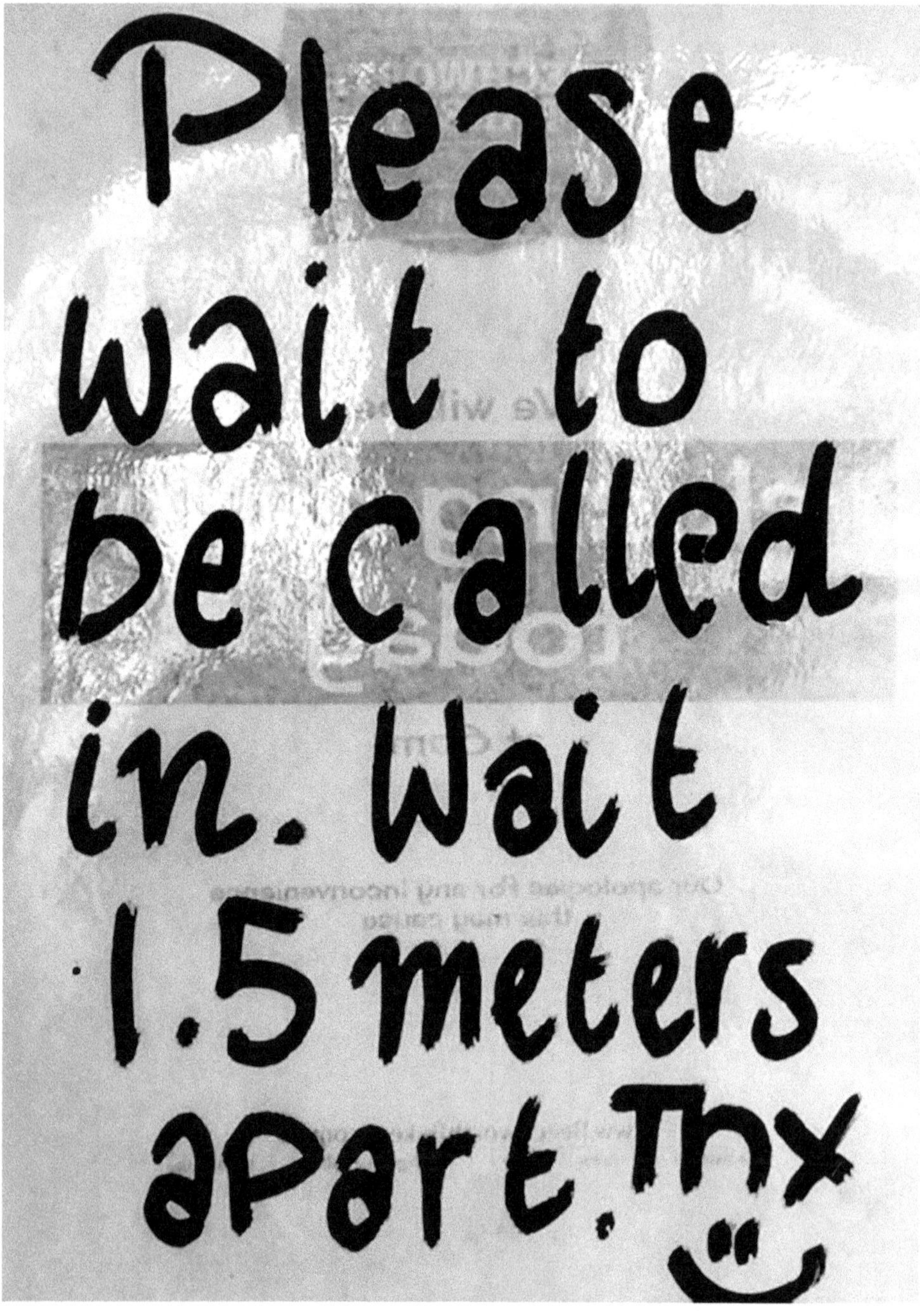
Please
wait to
be called
in. Wait
1.5 meters
apart. Thx

the bookfair is not described (in any text)

the bookfair
is not happening
this year

I was there
last year
manning a stall

fifteen thousand people
came

some bought a year's supply
of reading

thirteen books
in one purchase
and more
from other stalls

wow

but
the bookfair
in that little town
is not happening

crowds
of more than one hundred
are banned

and a lady said

> *we're closing down*
>
> *the whole town*
> *is about to die*

the new illnesses
are *depression*
and *despair*

the town's main street
is wide
from edge to edge

it was created
I think
in the days
of u-turning
horse-drawn wagons
a century ago

and it seems
as vast
as a wheat field

as empty
as the moon

and the pages
of no book
have been written
to describe it

something else (with cheesecake)

the café
is a chattering crowd

tables full

staff running
off their feet

small children
everywhere

the sun
is shining

maybe tomorrow
this will all
be banned

meanwhile

have a bite
of my cheesecake

this coffee
is divine

no

no
I mean *it*

today
let's talk
about something else

trust (judgement)

there comes a point
I suppose
in every crisis

where the names
of the leaders
matter

the nation's leaders

the world's leader

their identities
roll through the mind
in a wondering way
during the dark
of the middle
of the night

the names that
in these blackest hours
of our times
we need to trust –
implicitly
and completely –
to know what to do

we need to know
that *they*
want nothing more
than to do *right*
and to do *best*
by their people
now so dependent
upon them

trump
johnson
putin
xi

morrison
ardern
trudeau

rouhani and khamanei

kim

dhoni

merkel
macron

the names
that carry our trust
and our hope
in this time
of crisis

history
will judge

no doubt
no doubt

and perhaps –
in a small way –
I will judge
as well

defiance (and survival)

it was

unacceptable

that
is what the politicians
said

thousands of people
gathered
in defiance
on *bondi beach*
and failing to exercise
social distancing

the price
of disobeying
an edict
and official request
is the closure
of beaches

~

it was

unacceptable

that's what
the beach-lovers
said

they can't stop people
from living
like people

they can't be allowed
to impose fear
by decree

the over-reaction
is outrageous

and
just who
do they think
they are
to close down
our beach

~

it is

unacceptable . . .

is what the lady
walking her dog –
a little agitatedly –
on a strip of pavement
said

it is unacceptable
that a person
cannot walk alone
on the beach

at a time of such
distress
and isolation
and loneliness

a walk
beside water . . .

the feeling
of sand
between the toes . . .

but
the idiots
have shut down
the beach

all
of the beaches

why is it
that only the fools
survive

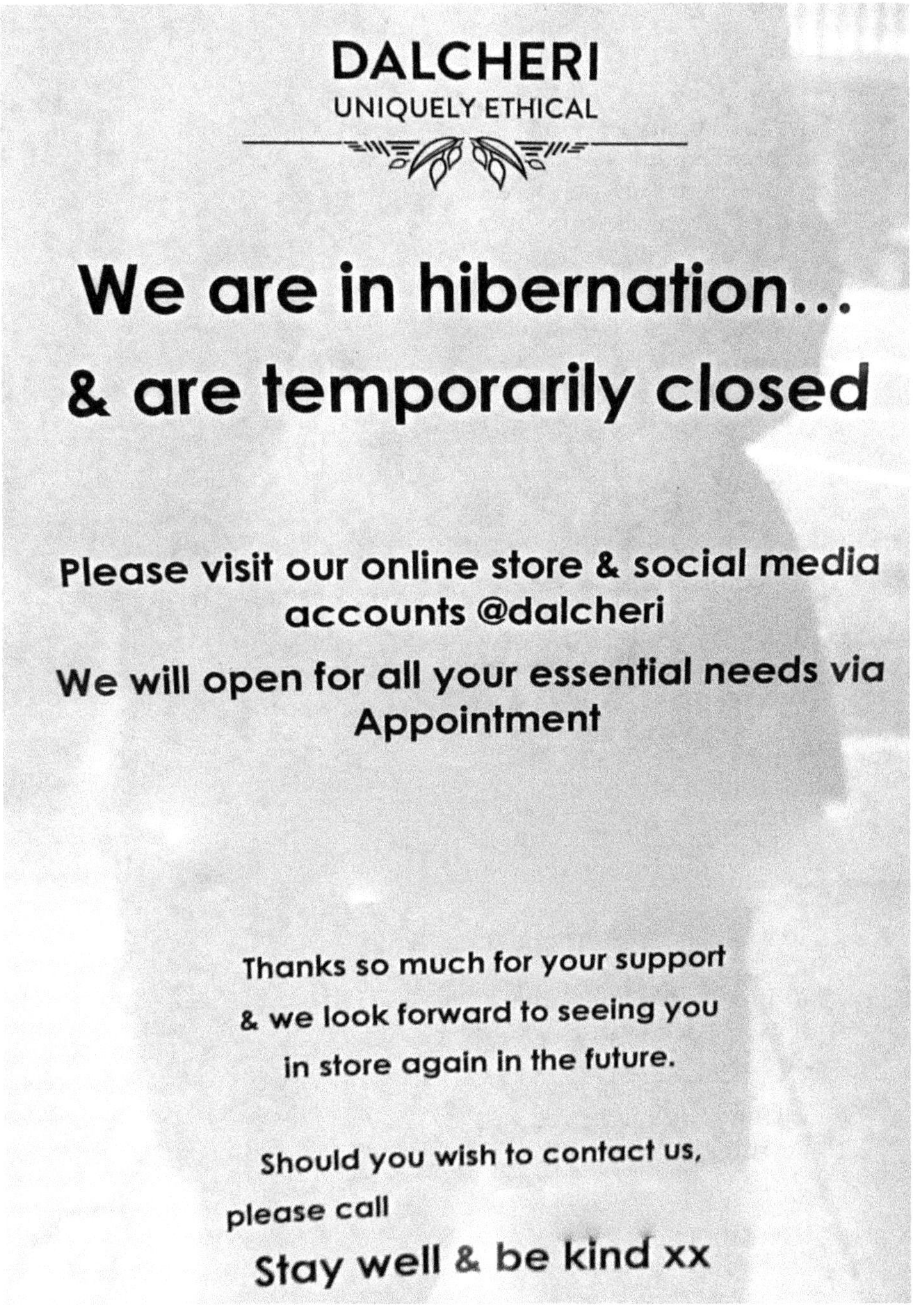
DALCHERI
UNIQUELY ETHICAL
We are in hibernation...
& are temporarily closed
Please visit our online store & social media accounts @dalcheri
We will open for all your essential needs via Appointment
Thanks so much for your support
& we look forward to seeing you
in store again in the future.
Should you wish to contact us,
please call
Stay well & be kind xx

an epoch (in a face mask)

not so long ago
we used to argue
about women
who covered up their faces
each time they left the house

never showed themselves
in public

some said
it shouldn't be allowed

some said
it was the sure sign
of a terrorist
lurking inside
a long dress

then
the summer of burning came
and smoke
filled up all our air

we couldn't see
a hand
held in front
of our faces

so we began wearing
masks
just to be able to breathe
if we needed to step
outside

we'd never experienced
anything quite like it
at the time

some thought . . .

and *I* thought
the world
might be coming to an end

and maybe it was

afterwards
we had a few good days
with clean air

and started to feel
as though life –
real life –
was on the way back

then
the virus came
and breathed all over
the whole
of the world

~

today
the government announced
that it expected the arrival
of about thirty-four million
face masks
within a week

so many

this time around
the air looks fine

it's clear and clean
but
it can make you sick

or kill you

the whole country
is sick

and it looks
to be dying

~

it was only
a very little while ago
we used to worry
about women
who covered their faces

that seems
such an epoch
in the past

a flash (to the end) of isolation

last night
the stars
were still up
in the sky

I stood awhile
just to watch them

bright spots
in the darkness

just
as they have
always been

it is infinite
up there

no end
and no beginning

just the flash
from a passing
meteor

shooting star
shooting star
can you see
all the way
to tomorrow
from up there

would you tell me
if you did

somehow
I don't think so

no *virus*
no *sickness*
no *welfare line*

no
stay at home

or
do not mingle

> *shooting star*
> *come back again*
> *for me*
>
> *I would ride*
> *with you to the end*
> *of such unsocial*
> *isolation*

weep (and pray) alone

there is weeping
as the shutters
close

another small café
is deemed
non-essential

no hotels
except bottle-shops

no restaurants
only
takeaway

no more
folk
than one hundred

no hugging
closer to the public street
than the length
of your driveway

no religion
except to wed

except to bury

so
find a way
and a place

by yourself

for your prayers
and your tears

may you find
release
in your weeping

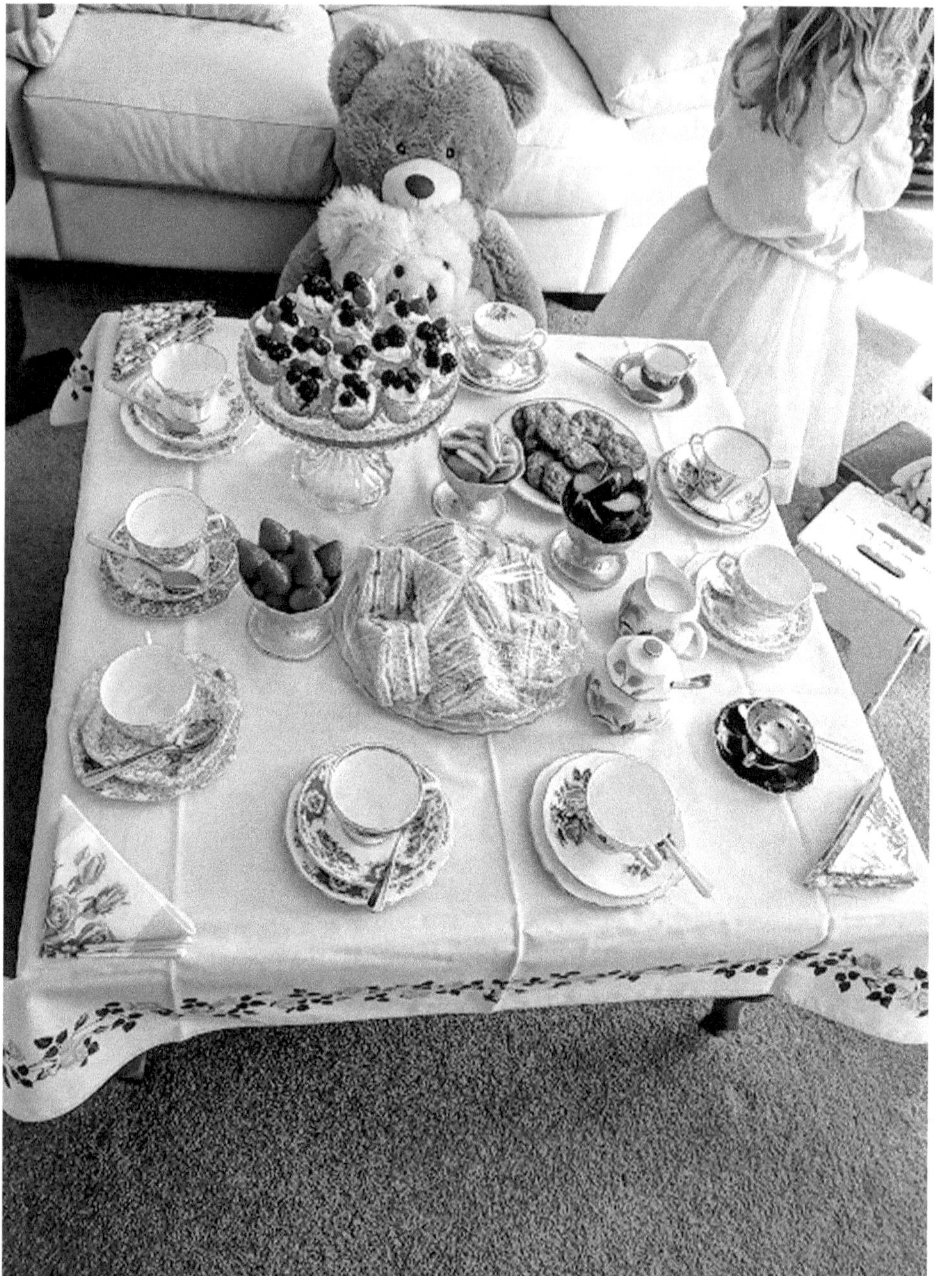

the future (is a child at play)

I was going
to write
again
about the shutdown
of everything considered
non-essential

but instead
as I contemplate
restriction
and the requirement
for life events –
long planned –
to be cancelled

I am distracted
by thoughts of the pleasure
that can come
with company

of how small children
represent something

unbridled *life*

and joy
even amidst incidental
tears

~

I was watching
today
a young boy
a small girl
at play

surrounded by adults
who had moved mountains
to create
a happy moment

a particular happy moment
in the course
of the day

so much laughter
from adult and child
both

and learning

for
the preparation of
a *high tea*
with the special presence
of teddy bears
is no small thing
to master

time spent with a child
in such circumstance
is surely
surely
the very *point*
of any future
that might be left to us

is it not

karen's story (as heard in the welfare line)

I was the last one
to be employed

it was my third job
working in
hospitality

but I
was the first one
to get the call

a quiet
sad word
from the manager

first to go

and now
all three jobs
are gone

I've got no money
but
the mortgage
is due
tomorrow

so far I haven't had a call
to say
that it's likely
to be waived

and I don't want
to cry about myself
I'm not the only one
like this

it's everyone
and
everywhere

but
I don't know
what I
am going to do . . .

and this line
to get the dole
moves slow

I'm not going –
not getting –
anywhere

.

.

.

my little girls
still need
to eat

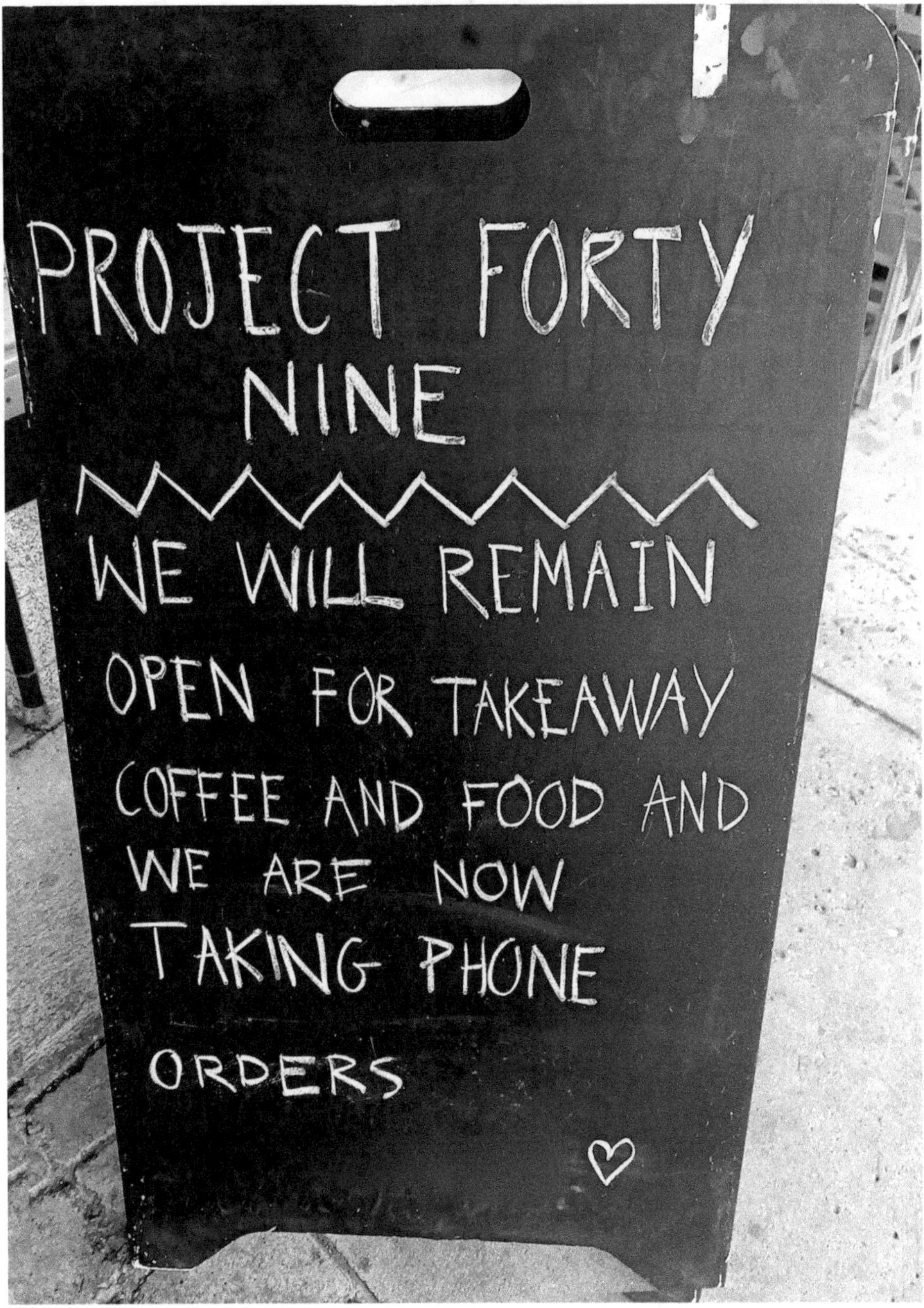
PROJECT FORTY
NINE
WE WILL REMAIN
OPEN FOR TAKEAWAY
COFFEE AND FOOD AND
WE ARE NOW
TAKING PHONE
ORDERS

fourteen years (out of picture)

there is a weeping
on the tv tonight

a man
closing down
his life
of the last fourteen years

a business
built from scratch

he can't
hold it together
on camera
as he tells his anguish
at having to
let go
his staff

his wonderful staff

and swearing
a vow
to start over again
when this virus . . .

this

this
disaster

is gone

day one
of year one
of
another fourteen

I'm sorry

he apologises to viewers

I'm sorry

turns away
to weep
into his hands
and out
of picture

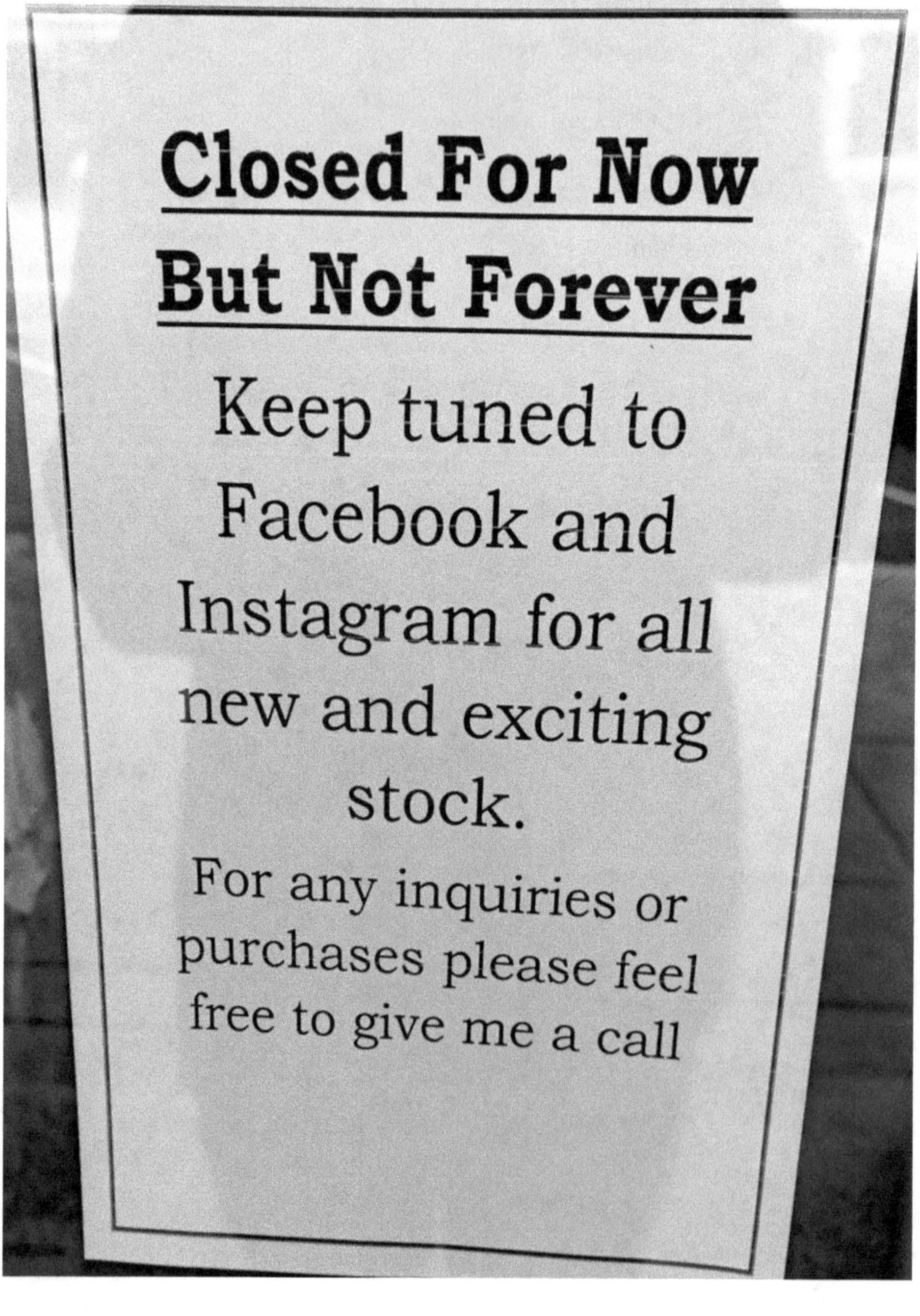
Closed For Now
But Not Forever
Keep tuned to
Facebook and
Instagram for all
new and exciting
stock.
For any inquiries or
purchases please feel
free to give me a call

a social distancing (of money)

at the hardware
store

at the butchery

there is black tape
marking out crosses
on the floor

they are placed a metre
and a half
apart

a sign
on the counter
declares

> *there is only room*
> *for three people*
> *at a time*
> *in this store*

responsible
social distancing
at work

at the bank
as I stepped
a pace forward
toward the glass

the teller
moved one pace
back

she gestured me
to return behind *my* line
so that *she*
could approach the counter
to do her work

a strange
and almost graceful
social distance dance

when I bought
a packet of seed
for the rejuvenation
of the home garden
the girl asked me
pleasantly
to please present the packets
with the barcode facing up
to facilitate scanning

and so that
she didn't have to touch
the packet
after I had handled it

pay by card

your money is no good
here
anymore

notice (the reef)

don't think
that I haven't noticed

the coral
of the great barrier reef
has been bleached
again

I can't say
it is the fault
of the virus

can't say
it has anything
to do
with the drought

or the fires

I can't say
but . . .

don't think for a moment
that I haven't
noticed

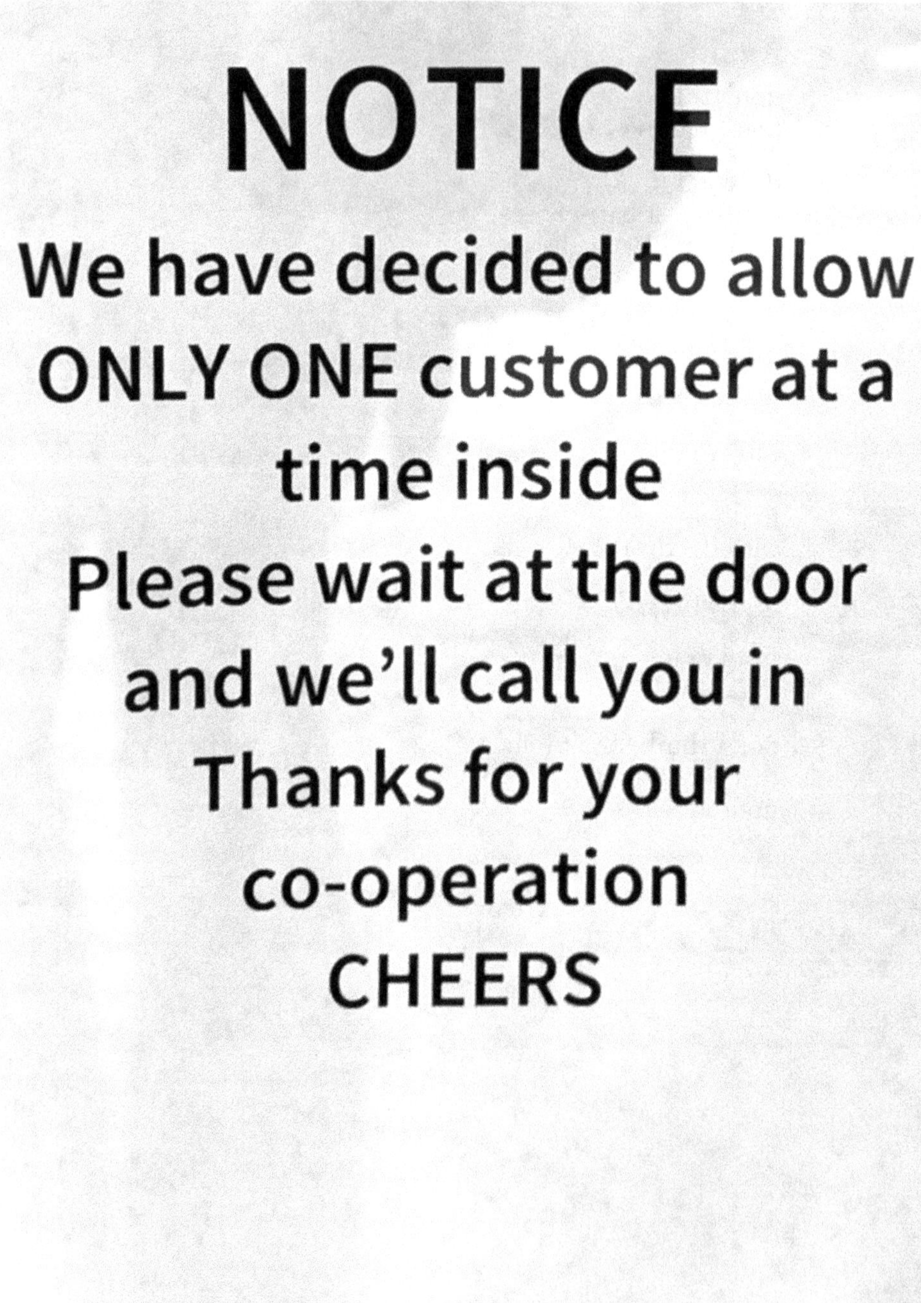
NOTICE
We have decided to allow
ONLY ONE customer at a
time inside
Please wait at the door
and we'll call you in
Thanks for your
co-operation
CHEERS

wishing a star (at four ay-em)

the stars
at four ay-em
are pinpoints
against the dark

but
I crane my neck
to watch them

a slow drift
of stellar cloud
sailing
the cosmos

indifferent
to small lives
and awe

but
a wish upon
is still
a wish upon

no matter the likelihood
of
my wish upon
being noticed
or attended

and I wished
upon a shooting light
that flashed by
peripherally

I turned my *want*
into a small request
and now
I hold it close

will it come true . . .

how
am I
to know

but
I closed my eyes
in the prescribed way
and wished my wish
with all my heart

that is all
that I
know how to do

I sent it
up
into the stellar night
a tiny hope
of mine

then turned back
inside
and
returned to bed

the shining stars
of four ay-em
within me

on (to the positive)

even I
sometimes
seek the positive

in the midst
of the train-wreck
that our lives have experienced

have *become*

in all the messy dismantling
of who and what
we've thought we are
that grows
and grows
daily

until
there seems no respite
from devastation

.

.

.

I seek
the optimistic

I find . . .

the silence

I find
the song of dawn
when I wake
still wondering
from a portentous dream

already fading

I find
the small
of me

the *little*

and
I find it
strong

I find
your presence

I am not
really
alone

you and I
are
a world
complete

and
in our way
we will go on

we will
go
on

b & b (no chance)

does anyone know

he asked
his local social media
contacts

the address
and the owner's details
of all
the air-b-&-b places

the short term
accommodation
in the town

we need
to check up
on them

to make damn sure
no one
is renting them
over easter

no one should be allowed
to use them
for a holiday

no one

a reply came

if you're that
concerned
you better make sure
you stay at home
yourself

reflection (of the sacrifice)

easter

resurrection comes

but before that
I must die

or so
I understand . . .

I wonder

how does that work

but
I doubt
that I need to know

it is a matter
of the soul

perhaps
of the underworld

and I am willing
enough
if it is
for the good

for the *very* good
and
for us all

I look around

and I have to stare
at what
I see

at what
is left

a cannibal
to eat the moon

darkness
for night

what has happened
to the day I knew
before

symbols abound

symbols
inform

the old mother
is suffering
in her own distress

the ferocity
of storms
should tell some part
of the tale

the contagion
running through my veins

through *all*
veins
is like the fear
that imposes itself
now

it is each of us

kept alone
and sequestered
from what we know

from what we knew

from what we
assumed
in arrogance

just like our hope

kept far away
now
and safely distant

perhaps
this time . . .

this eastertime
we *all* have to die
in our own
little ways

perhaps –
yes –
to resurrect
but . . .

I wonder
what will be
should I rise

should we all
rise

again

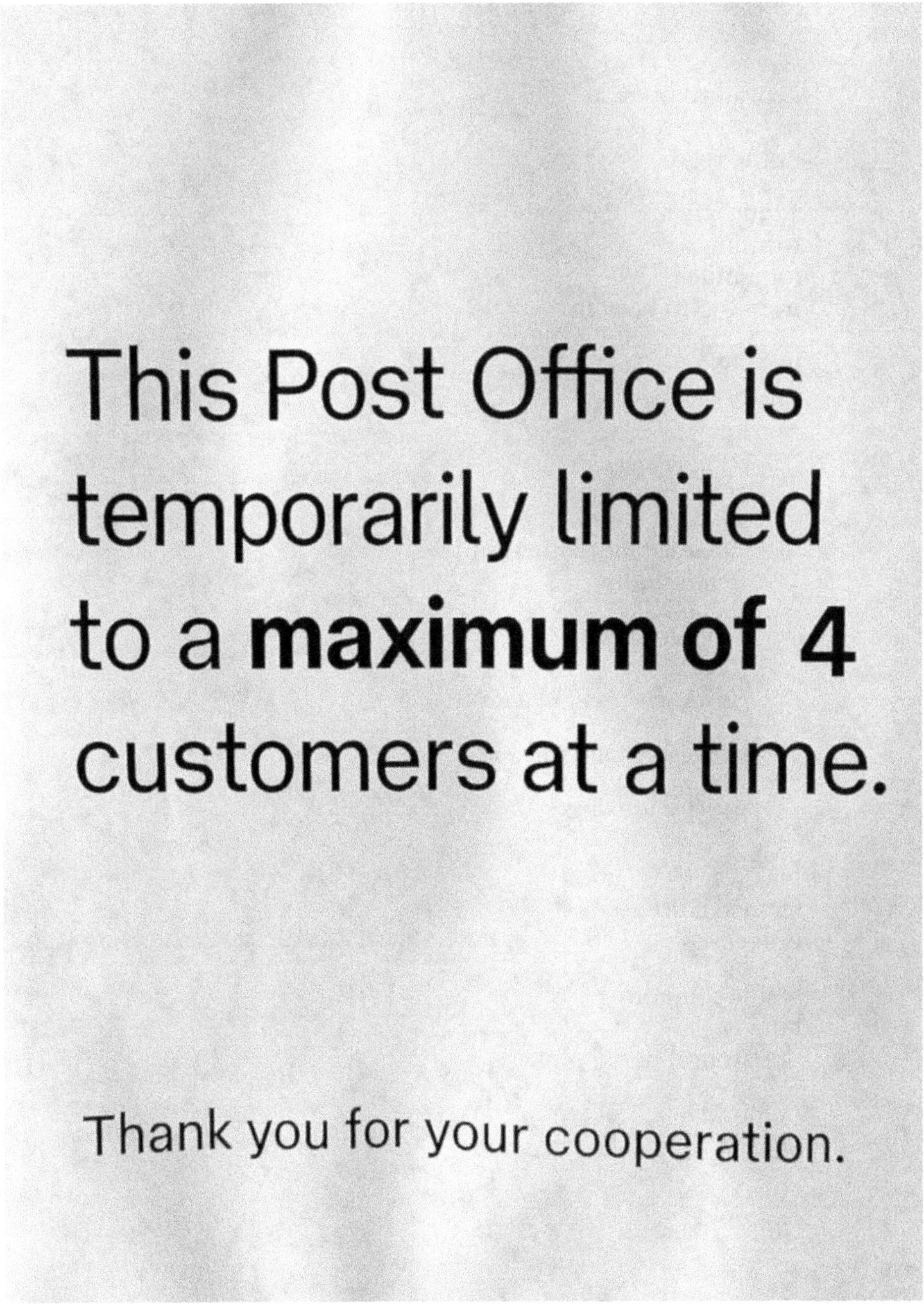
This Post Office is temporarily limited to a **maximum of 4** customers at a time.
Thank you for your cooperation.

a scream (no it was nothing really)

he walked outside
to the centre
of the road

a long street
running
for a mile
from top to bottom

usually
a busy one

trucks and cars

tankers diverting
to avoid the beating heart
of the town

timber trucks
laden
with sawlogs of radiata

tradies zooming around

people walking

his eyes
seemed a little
unfocused

seeing something
but
not around here

not anywhere
nearby

and not close enough
to notice
that he was wearing nothing
but his underpants

jockey briefs
in the bikini cut

he wobbled
a little

unsteady
on his feet
or perhaps
standing on a stone

it can be hard
to tell
exactly what is *wrong*
when a person
is in such
discomfort

if
there was anyone
to *see*

anyone
to *say*

but
he was alone

no traffic
today

just like
there was no traffic
yesterday

silence

until he raised
his head

perhaps his eyes
came into focus then

perhaps not

identification of
just what is
in focus
when a person
is in
such discomfort
can prove to be
a challenge

and he screamed

a long
drawn-out
wail
of a scream

it projected

anguish

and

dismay

and

loneliness

emptiness

pointlessness

loss
of hope

loss
of belief

loss
of everything

the cry
echoed
down
and up
the canyon of the street

and he finally
closed his eyes

sagged a little
then turned
and hobbled
away

back inside
the house

.

.

.

across the road
just for a moment
it *seemed* as though
a curtain
had twitched

as though –
maybe –
someone
had heard
something

in isolation (welcome welcome)

there is
a kind of peace
to the good days
of isolation

the sky is a mix of cloud
and blue

sunshine falls
here
and there

and here

and there

sound
is just a cockatoo

a distant dog

the patter
of my fingers
finding the keyboard
to write this note
that I intend
for you

wherever you are

I wish you
a soundbite
of my magpie

carolling the day

I wish you
the flight
of my butterfly
wandering
across the yard

I wish you
the green
that is my grass

my lawn

it looks alive
and growing
even as I watch

and
I wish you
a touch
from the breeze
that just now
brushed my face
on this
isolation day

welcome
to my
isolation day

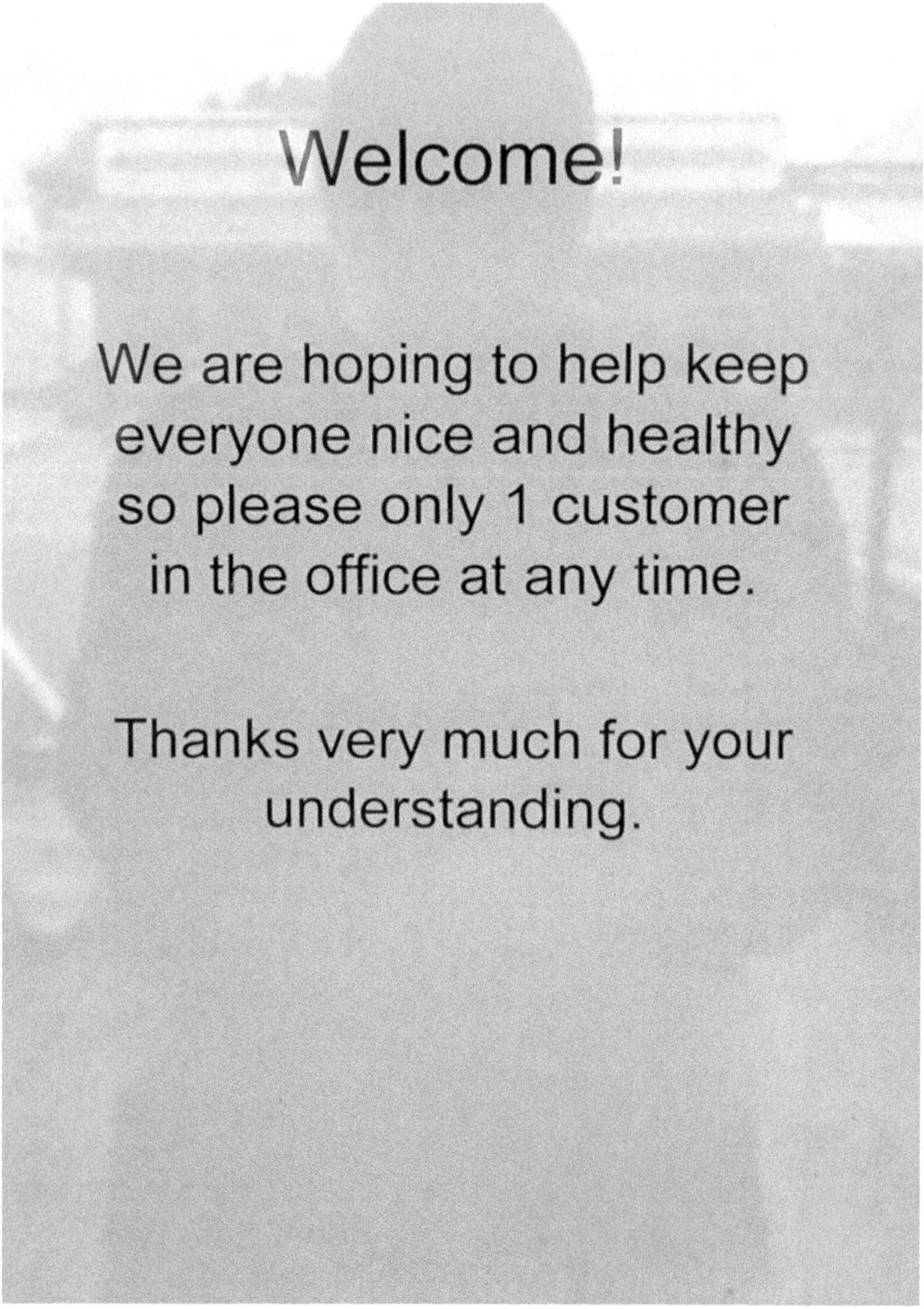
Welcome!
We are hoping to help keep everyone nice and healthy so please only 1 customer in the office at any time.
Thanks very much for your understanding.

never again (pariah)

I know
where you were

and I know
who you were with

is it any wonder
that you catch
such things

are you surprised
at all
that you've been
brought
so low

(*you know*)
I only watch
to keep you safe

to keep you close
and
within my loving gaze

.

.

.

there

you
have been out
again

I can see the signs
all over you
so
don't say a word

don't
excuse yourself

you know
and *I know* well
that
if you don't stop

next time
it will be
the strap

it will be
a punishment

a new name

I will call you
pariah

I do this
with
only love

with
all my love
and all my *heart*
for you

but
I *know*
where you've been

and you
must not go there
ever
again

https://www.theguardian.com/australia-news/2020/may/15/covid-safe-app-australia-how-download-does-it-work-australian-government-covidsafe-covid19-tracking-downloads

ganache and old candles (and zoom)

she said:

it was a birthday

an eighteenth
birthday
but
I couldn't buy flour
anywhere
to bake a cake

just the week before
I had to hunt all over
for icing

but no
so I made a ganache
instead

cream
for the whipping
was found –
somehow
from somewhere –
and we dredged up
some pre-loved
candles

it was special
I suppose
because
you only turn adult
the once

and there were her friends –
the guests –
all of them

lined up
across the screen
in row
upon row

no gifts from stores
and all non-essentials
banned

so
it was just us
in the room
and the best
we could do

her friends
everywhere

ganache
and old candles
and a session
on live-stream

happy birthday
dear one

happy birthday
to you

maybe
in a year

a better year
we can do it
again

next time
to feel
real

a star (unwrit)

one
by one

the stars
will fall

though they seem
so many
in the sky

a wink

a nod

and another light
out

it will be
all dark
by and by

but the night
doesn't seem
to notice

the night
goes on

without care

and it never –
not once –
stops to ask
perhaps
why

another line
remains silent

another line
unwritten
by *hand*

just
another all-too-disposable
pen

with ink
now allowed
to run dry

a remembering

april 25th
is anzac day
in australia

once every year
folk gather
to remember
the ones
that didn't come home
from a war

or didn't come home
the same
as
when they left

red poppies
at dawn . . .

this year
that can't be done

the virus
is a war
all its own

so *this* year
a trumpet sounds
in the darkness

and people stand
on the street
in front
of their houses

and light candles in the window
right beside
a row of medals
or a ribbon

and somehow
the feeling
of a sacred moment
is shared

the self-isolation
of a nation
gets broken down
one person
at a time

by a moment held
in unison
at the end of the driveway

or
standing on the lawn

and a minute
of silence

It is with great sadness that Beechworth G has decided to close to the public.

If you need to pick up a layby, have a courier drop off, or would like to purchase something gorgeous, please call for assistance.

We wish you and your families a safe few months ahead.

Cook beautiful meals every day, do some exercise, look up how to "Prancercise" for a giggle, don't forget to call all the people you love for a chat.

Be strong and brave, we will get through this!

And we can't wait to see all your gorgeous faces again soon.

All Our Love

Beechworth G

tp (at eight) and meaningful data

the local store
sent a note out
on social media:

we've got TP
on the shelf

there's a limit
for each customer

and
we're not going to open
the doors
at seven ay-em
anymore

nobody's been coming in
so you
can come by
at eight

just like
in normal times

normal times
these days
are spent
staring at the garden

it is green
with the rain
and growing about as fast
as life moves

about as fast
as I move
in my bedroom slippers
at half-past
the day

the government
has an application –
an *app* –
they want me
to download

they think
they will see
who I have mingled with
if I happen to get unwell

but . . .

I don't know

the way that *I*
seem to socialise
these days
it could be a long
lonesome
wait

for meaningful data

unknowing (the city)

the trees
do not care
beyond yellow
and red

the stream
does not worry
it just runs

for the rains
have come
and the world
has turned

it is autumn again
as it should be

the city –
close by –
has died
just a little

and there is trouble
now
in finding
a soul

for it is people
that it *needs*
and the people
are all afraid
inside their homes

nothing
is on the streets
but their echo

and a little
lost
paper-litter
that rides on a wind
whose song is sung
quite alone

but the trees
around my village
don't live
a city life

they feel
for the changes
in the air

for the colour
in their leaves
as one season
becomes the next

and
if people stay home
they don't know it

if the city
is alone
the trees
are not aware

it could be (as a vow)

it occurs to me
belatedly

it could come for me

it is a virus
hungry and voracious

I
am just a man
like any other

like any other
victim
not yet confirmed
to be like
a *survivor*

I feel myself invincible
but also vulnerable

both feelings
in rapid succession

and at the same time

unseeing
and yet surrounded

the statistics . . .

the dying
are just numbers

the people
that they might have been
are random

unknown by me

~

Closed For Now

my outing

my daily outing
to the supermarket
for one of *this*
some
of *that*

my walk
stepping wide to avoid
a passing human being

my waking breath . . .

anything that I do

anywhere
that I am

.

.

.

every breath
that I take
could be the one

the *introduction*

the virus
may like me

it may settle

it might take me
in a marriage
to itself

for ever

until death
do
us

the door (of numbers)

I have become
fascinated
by the numbers

the *united states* numbers

in my morning
in
their night

a thousand . . .

fifteen hundred . . .

less today

more again
tomorrow

from where
comes the courage
to step outside
the door

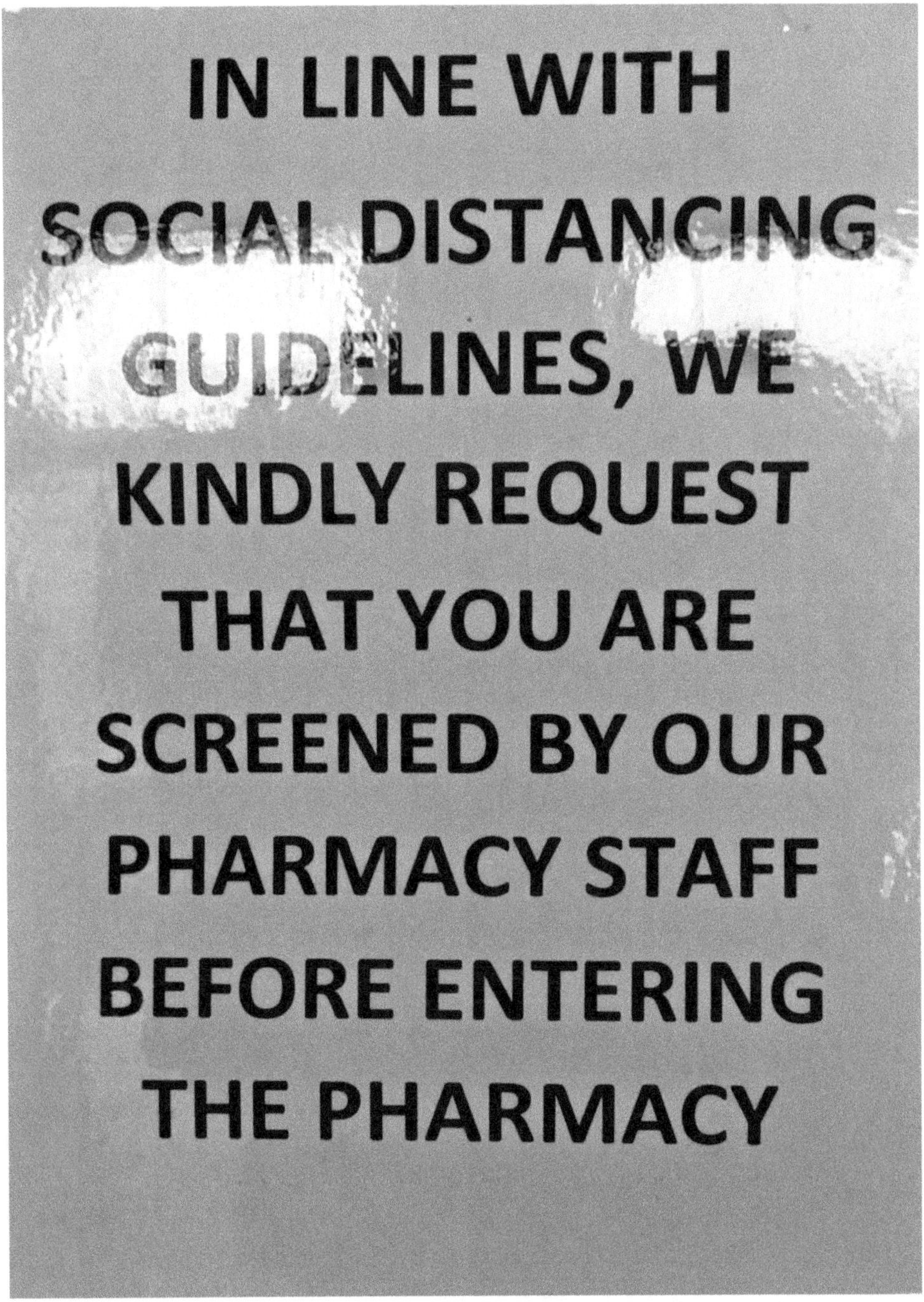
IN LINE WITH
SOCIAL DISTANCING
GUIDELINES, WE
KINDLY REQUEST
THAT YOU ARE
SCREENED BY OUR
PHARMACY STAFF
BEFORE ENTERING
THE PHARMACY

Part II: The Facility

entrance

the way in
is via automatic doors
at the entrance to the short stay
acute section
but
the doors do not open
automatically
anymore

first
it is necessary
to confront an intercom

nurses
on the other side
have now become
portal-keepers
and interrogators

they ask the same questions
of every visitor
on every visit

> *have you been keeping*
> *bad company*
>
> *have you been*
> *in foreign climes*
>
> *have you coughed*
> *run a temperature*
> *found it hard to breathe*

it doesn't matter
that they have asked him already
yesterday
and the day before

through the inner doors

do not pass
the handwash station
uncleansed

then
along corridors
to reach the internal entrance
of the long-stay area

the facility

a friendly staff
show genuine pleasure
at greeting another visitor

he has encountered them
before
at shift handover
and cannot help
but wonder
at the impossibility
of maintaining social separation
when there are eight nurses
crammed
into one
small
nurses' station

visiting

the old man
is sitting
in a chair beside the bed
in his room

his upper body is covered
but his legs
are bare

patterned
with reddening lines
that suggest
they are cold

he makes a gesture
to suggest
it is of no concern

mumbles a story
of nurses
and breakfasts

of routine
interrupted

but mostly
of nothing *mattering*
anymore

it will not be long
the old man suggests
until *nothing*
will matter
anymore

the daily newspapers
are open
on the bedside table
as they always are

his days now
spent pondering
the news
between the regular
interruptions

morning tea

lunch

a nap

maybe a little exercise
or a quiz
at some point

the headlines scream

coronavirus

and he is
genuinely
puzzled

disconcerted
in his attempts
to take in the magnitude
of this new scourge
that is loose
in the world

to comprehend
the changed reality
raging
just beyond his doors

shakes his head

at the outlandishness
of what he is reading

the idea
that is self-isolation

at people hoarding
toilet paper

a million workers
newly unemployed . . .

in this *country*

but the look
in his eyes
becomes tearful
when he asks for a clarification

is it true

could it *possibly*
be *true*
that only ten mourners
will be allowed to attend
his funeral
if he dies

exit

for the son
leaving at the end of the visit
feels
almost like stepping into
springtime

there is a sense
of needing to run
through the corridors
to achieve the outside

to be bathed
in sunshine
with no other soul
to be seen

no sound
to be heard

the moment
of embrace
by unsullied air
is a giant step
away
from an atmosphere
of subdued oppression

it remains necessary
to self-isolate
back to his home

and then
adjust mentally
to the fact that
the relative peace
and tranquillity there
is now a legislated requirement

but the illusion
of normality
is *almost* easy

almost
straightforward

until *the news hour*
and fresh reports
of additional
imposed restrictions

when –
in the back of his mind –
he finds himself wondering
if he will be able to locate
as *many* as ten
available mourners
when the old man's time
has come

unless (for palliation)

it has taken
a while

the old man
and his son
have developed a relationship
that has certain
unspoken
rules

the old man
has always been competent
in areas where the son
has not

skilled artisan work
performed by hand
and general labouring
are the old man's skill set

his sense of personal control
and competence
has always been
vital
to him

the son knows
to step
across thresholds

break through boundaries

there has been
a gradual transition
in the relativities
of relationship

and
as the old man's abilities
have diminished
and frailties
emerged
so the son
has gradually had to assume
more responsibilities
on his behalf

it is a
largely unspoken
transition

visitation
at the facility is
a mostly silent affair
that strives
to achieve an atmosphere
of genial co-tolerance

the conclusion is always a question
and answer
routine

are there any things
that you need

any tasks or chores
that will not wait

bills
to be paid

lately
health has begun
to fail

frailty has encroached
and the ability
of the old man
to leave his room . . .

to leave his oxygen
supply . . .

the ability
to be larger than life
in the usual ways . . .

has abandoned him

his interests
have diminished
proportionately
and conversation
is now more likely to focus
on joining
his deceased wife
underground
than
to do with living

there has been talk
among concerned staff
that older folk –
even less physically compromised
than the old man –
may well succumb
to the lack of hope and prospect
that pervades all activities
now

they are concerned that
he may
just
give up

at the most recent visit
though
there was an apparent change

a sense
that he appreciated the presence
of the younger man . . .

of his son

and that the atmosphere
between them
was —
perhaps —
becoming genuinely
appreciated

awaited

acknowledged

it is a new
small pleasure
for them both

~

today
there is a phone call
from the facility

> *due*
> *to the pandemic*
> *no further visits*
> *will be allowed*
>
> *unless*
> *for palliation*

all visits are cancelled
for the good

> *for the greater good*

of us all

searching (for air)

the sheer curtain
rises

and falls

a soft billowing
as though
the other side
is a place
of whispers

of summonses

and an apparent response
is *gasped*
aloud

breath
by struggled breath

the rapid
stuttering movement
of the coverlet
is evidence
of the toll
such conversation demands

hush now
hush

morphine
and *midaz*

hush awhile

breathe easy

there is nothing
in the world

nothing
at the end

beyond the search –
desperate
and dire –
for air

for one

next

breath

of air

conveying (by hand)

last night
the old man's hand
was warm
to the touch

it was a night
for holding
though
in these times
of rampant virus
it seems sometimes
that touch
requires the issuance
of a licensed permission

this morning
though
the hand is cool

and
the son
holds it

gives
a squeeze

receives

.

.

.

a squeeze

gently rubs a finger
over
a finger

if it is possible
to convey
through touch
what is being felt
emotionally
then . . .

the son
conveys
all
that is possible

about an ending (in seventeen syllables)

do you wonder
about the end
of life

it is labour

hard
labour

almost gone (is the day)

the son sits
patiently

watches the bed

a jerking
abruptness
forms itself
into a rhythm
that then becomes
each individual breath

an oxygen mask –
initially placed carefully
over the old man's face –
is displaced

again and again

by the vigour
of his efforts
in pursuit of air

again
and again

the mask travels north
toward
the eyes

that
is ambition
for you

morphine

is an angel

is a blanket

is a shroud

morphine descends

.

.

.

let all troubles
subside

.

.

.

the son
thinks his own thoughts

I
am a day

life
is a year
that is gone

almost . . .

gone

he studies the jerkiness
of breathing
on the bed

almost
almost
gone

a drift (behind clouds)

the son is evicted
so the nurses can do
what nurses do

people . . .

staff of the facility

stop
to talk

always

usually
keeping to the required
distances and degrees
of separation

in these compromised times
they have begun
to grieve

it has become apparent
without the need
for speech
that *this* time
the vigil
will be final

and all question

> *what kind of a time*
> *is this*
> *for a man*
> *to die*
>
> *when the virus prevails*
> *to such an extent*
> *that only ten people*
> *can attend a funeral . . .*

including the celebrant
and the undertaker

how is it
that this sub-microscopic
wretch
of a disease-thing
can prevent loved ones . . .

a peep
through the door
reveals uniforms

and scrawny
naked legs

a groan
as the body is raised
into the air
on a hoist
to allow
a mattress change

to make the last part
of this journey
a little more comfortable

it is better
to stay outside

to find
a coffee-companion
for a waiting hour

another waiting day

all
that yet remains
of a life

drifting
like the sun
behind a cloud

uncomfortable sensation (a rattle on the bed)

the son watches
as they

put a line
in

let the morphine
run
as needed
instead of by injection
every two hours

the old man
will get relief
for his breathing

as–and–when
he requires it
now

watching
this struggle
to breathe
is becoming
unbearable

the son feels
an unaccustomed
emotion

and his stoic demeanour
in the role
of watcher
from the sidelines
is challenged
by the uncomfortable sensation
of a lump
in his throat

while all the while
the rattle
on the bed
is such very
very
demanding labour

a hospital song (in quiet voice)

the son sings
a hospital song

raises the voice
inside himself

makes it loud
even while he remains
outwardly silent

his tune is accompanied
by the rattle
of apparatus

the groan
of air

the muted call
of nurse
to nurse
on the far side
of the closed door

somebody laughs

he doesn't
really
hear them

he sings
in his silent voice
a hospital song

toward (fare well)

they ask if he agrees
on the old man's behalf
that they should administer

a little more

to ease
the battle
but . . .

you know that
a little more
might . . .

well

he contemplates

who can tell

life is chances
taken
choices made

and
a little ease toward
fare
well
should not be denied

summon now (weeks may pass)

yes

he is told

make the call

summon loved ones

this
can only conclude
one way
now

in these *corona* times
two weeks
of self-isolation
may need to pass
before any who must travel
can attend

and the sand
can only flow
until
the last grain
falls

until
there is no more

yes

he is told

call them
now

alone (after breath)

he noticed
the character
and sound
of the old man's breathing
change

from laboured
and stertorous

to soft

hesitant
with pauses

he noticed . . .

.

.

.

nothing

and was
quite suddenly
alone

the time (duly noted)

the man –
no longer *the younger*
but still
the son –
went to some small
trouble
to note the time . . .

the exact
minute

but afterwards
had to laugh
to himself

a little wryly

for he could not
remember
just when
the old man
had died

deeply (the quiet of a day)

outside

it felt like
forever
since he had last been
outside

in the daylight

it was necessary
to wash his hands
of course
for there is still
a pandemic
raging

but the quiet

> *the absence*
> *of stertor . . .*
>
> *the existence of cars*
>
> *and sounds*
>
> *and the very width*
> *and breadth*
> *of day . . .*

were experienced
as a wonder

he stood
with eyes closed
and drew a breath
deeply

silence (the day after)

it was the silence
that he noticed

lying in bed
at first light

silence

like a pool
of lamplight
and himself
within it

a boundary
and the sense
of day
not yet
begun

even the birds
chortling the morning
were
an incorporated part
of the quiet

he wondered
how silent . . .

could it be
more silent
beneath the ground

an idle wonder
though
and
of no consequence

the old man
was gone

buried

and
in his absence had come
this new sensation

of utter
silence

a visit (to drink the day)

the first return
to the family home –
delayed
until a mandatory period
of quarantine
due to the virus –
was meant to be
a *walk-through*

an appraisal
of what
was to be done

what cleared
what cleaned
what sold
what gifted

the death
and passing
had been . . .

what

soft
perhaps

uneventful

dignified

ease
at the last

the burial . . .

a simple thing
and sombre

sadly appropriate
for virus times

this visit
should have been
to view
emptiness
and to draw up
the plan
for dealing with it

a preliminary to
and a form of
last rites

but
each step
into the kitchen and bathroom
and bedrooms
and laundry
was somehow
lead-heavy
with the stale traces
of life

the workshops outside
and the shedding . . .

laden
with weight enough
to bow the spirit
of any would-be
tidier

an anticipatory garbage skip
filled to the brim
already
and awaiting removal
sounding
like a cry of anguish

rising
in crescendo
from everything
once important
but *now* . . .

just an inexplicable accumulation
of old *bits*
and of *bobs*

the outright sum
of *paraphernalia*
and *dross*
that comprised the totality
and meaning
of the old man
and his life

each step
an oppression

a desecration

dust entering
via slightly flared
nostrils
to impede any sense
of easy breathing

worse
in the imagination
than the reviled virus
itself

a personality
swathed and swirled

taking gradual shape
in the throbbing form
of a headache

this first return

the planned
easy
first visit

lingering
as a shape

a haunting
that absorbed entirely
all of the day
that remained

After Words

Author Information

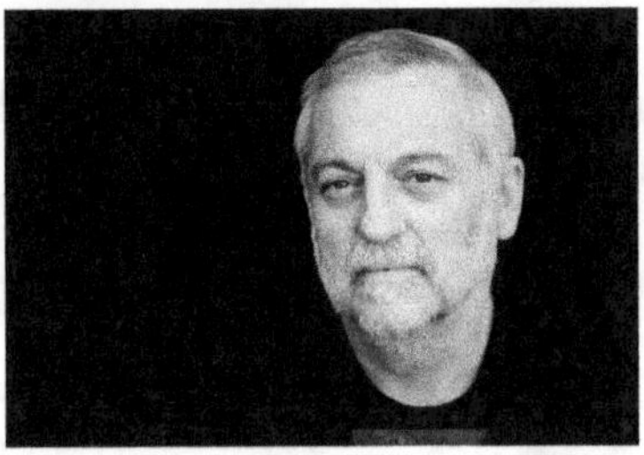

Frank Prem has been a storytelling poet since his teenage years. He has been a psychiatric nurse through all of his professional career, which now exceeds forty years.

He has been published in magazines, online zines, and anthologies in Australia, and in a number of other countries, and has both performed and recorded his work as spoken word.

Frank is an Adjunct Research Associate of the School of Education, Charles Sturt University, Australia.

He lives with his wife in the beautiful township of Beechworth in North East Victoria, Australia.

Connect with Frank

Find Frank at his website www.FrankPrem.com, or through Social Media online at Facebook, X (Twitter), Instagram and YouTube.

Other Published Works

Archive

A Poetry Archive – Volume 1 (2024)
A Poetry Archive – Volume 2 (2024)
A Poetry Archive – Volume 3 (2024)
A Poetry Archive – Volume 4 (2024)
A Poetry Archive – Volume 5 (2025)
A Poetry Archive – Volume 6 (2025)
A Poetry Archive – Volume 7 (2025)

Memoir

Small Town Kid (2018)
The New Asylum (2019)

Picture Poetry Series

Pilgrim Volume 1 - Illustrated by Leanne Murphy (2024)
A Lake Sambell Walk (2021)
A Few Places Near Home (2023)
The Unsuspected Slums (2026)
Write Places Write Times (2026)

Children's Picture Books

The Beechworth Bakery Bears (2021)
Waiting for Frank-Bear (2021)
On Allium Avenue (2025)

Bachelard Interpreted

A Choir of Whispers (2024).
A Cleansing Flame (2024)
Real Weight (2025)
A Flight Of Ideas (2025)
An Ocean of Purity (2025)
The Kiss Reverberant (2025)
Monet's Lily (2026)
Air To Breathe (2026)

Speculative Poetry

The Garden Black (2022)
A Specialist At The Recycled Heart (2022)
The Cielonaut (2024)

A Love Poetry Trilogy

Walk Away Silver Heart (2020)
A Kiss for the Worthy (2020)
Rescue and Redemption (2020)
Alive Is What You Feel (2023)

Natural Disasters

Devil In The Wind (2019)
Of Drought and Fire (2025)
SMALL Change (2025)
Closed For Now (2026)

War and Conflict

Sheep On The Somme (2021)
From Volyn To Kherson (2023)

Free Verse

Pebbles to Poems (2020)
White Whale (2024)
Ida: Searching for The Jazz Baby (2023)
Herja, Devastation With Cage Dunn (2019)

What Readers Say

Small Town Kid

A modern-day minstrel. Highly recommended.

–A. F. (Australia)

Small Town Kid is a wonderful collection.

–S. T. (Australia)

Devil In The Wind

Trust me, this book will stay with you. Bravo!

–K. K. (USA)

Moving, beautiful, and terrible. I was left with a profound sense of respect, as well as a reminder that we should never take for granted every precious every moment of life.

–J. S. (South Africa)

The New Asylum

Words can't do justice to the emotional journey I travelled in (reading this collection).

–C. D. (Australia)

If I had to pick one book over the past year that has truly resonated with me, this would be it.

–K. B. (USA)

Walk Away Silver Heart

Instantly grips you by the throat in his step-by-step story of survival. Bravo!

–K. K. (USA)

Outstanding!

–B. T. (Australia)

A Kiss For The Worthy

A Celebration of Life Written in Thoughtful Bursts of Poetic Expression

–C M C (United States)

With every verse, I found myself reflecting about myself, my life, and the world.

–K

Rescue and Redemption

The passion of love in its many forms explored by one for another.

–J L (United States)

I've enjoyed every word, every breath. Every moment within the life of these stories.

–C D (Australia)

Sheep On The Somme

Museums and archivists take note–sell this in your gift shops, preserve it in your archives. Professors, teachers–share with your students.

–A R C (United States)

(This) book is a beautiful and graphic tribute to all those brave men and women who gave their lives for their countries between 1914 and 1918.

–R C (South Africa)

Ida: Searching for The Jazz Baby

I found myself deeply moved by the presentation of Ida's elusive, illusionary life.

–E G (United States)

He gives her a depth and vulnerability that the press didn't.

– A C (United Kingdom

The Garden Black

Prem creates verse that illuminates our world, its experiences and history.
–S C (United Kingdom)

Prem's poetry reminds that life is fragile and fleeting ... both harsh and beautiful.
–D G K (Canada)

A Few Places Near Home

The author has captured many beautiful images in this book, and is a wonderful photographer as well as a poet. This book would make a beautiful coffee table book filled with moving prose to make us ponder with gorgeous accompanying images.
–D K (Canada)

www.FrankPrem.com

www.ingramcontent.com/pod-product-compliance
Lightning Source LLC
LaVergne TN
LVHW022033200926
848481LV00007B/2674
* 9 7 8 1 9 2 5 9 6 3 1 3 7 *